The Calorie Count Method:
With Delicious Chicken Recipes

Choosing sensible portions is a key to controlling calorie intake and getting or keeping your weight in a healthy range. The Calorie Count Method helps you stay on track with managing your weight.

Knowing one's daily calorie needs may be a useful reference point for determining whether the calories that a person eats and drinks are appropriate in relation to the number of calories needed each day. The Calorie Count Method is a simple solution to what may be a difficult problem.

Table of Contents

How Many Calories Do You Eat?

Suppose you had dinner at an Italian restaurant last night. You ordered spaghetti with meatballs. While you were waiting for your order, you ate 2 slices of garlic bread. How can you tell if this dinner is too much food for you? You should estimate how much you ate and then compare that to the Food Guide Pyramid recommendations.

Think about your plateful of spaghetti and meatballs. Then estimate the amounts of spaghetti, sauce, and meat. You may decide, for example, that the spaghetti portion was about 2 cups, the tomato sauce looked like about 1 cup, and the meatballs were about 6 ounces. With the 2 slices of garlic bread, you now have an idea about how much you ate for dinner. But how do your portions translate into standard servings?

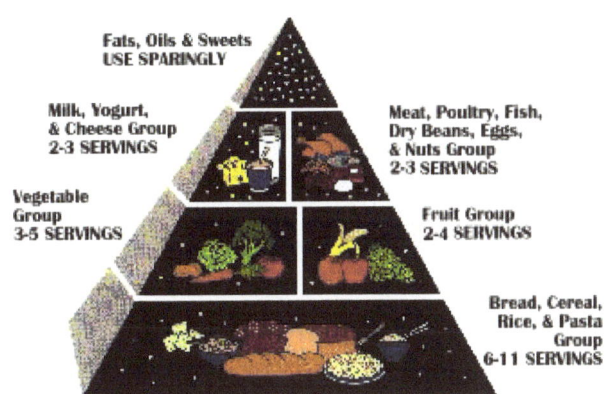

Pyramid Recommendations

To figure out if your spaghetti dinner was the right amount of food for you, use the Pyramid. Over a day, you should plan on eating the number of servings recommended from each group.

For example, if you need about 1,600 calories a day, the Pyramid recommends 6 daily servings from the Grains (Bread, Cereal, Rice & Pasta) group. How does this compare to your spaghetti dinner?

Your dinner had 6 servings—the total daily recommendation for someone with your calorie needs. If you had counted your portions of spaghetti and bread as only1 serving each, you might think you had only eaten 2 servings from the Grains group. But, you actually ate 6! By comparing the portion you ate with a standard Pyramid serving, you can judge whether your daily intake is right for you. Pyramid serving sizes and the recommended number of servings from each group are guides to help determine your daily intake.

Your portions do not have to match the standard serving size—they can be larger or smaller. But, the amount you eat over the day should match the total amount of a food that is recommended. Often, the food portions of grains and meats that people choose are larger than the Pyramid serving size. Be especially careful when counting servings from these groups to figure out how many Pyramid servings are in your portions.

The number of servings from each food group recommended by the Pyramid depends on your calorie needs.

• Children ages 2 to 6 years, many inactive women, and some older adults may need about 1,600 calories per day.
• Most children over 6, teen girls, active women, and many inactive men may need about 2,200 calories per day.
• Teen boys and active men may need

For example, if you need about 1,600 calories a day, the Pyramid recommends 6 daily servings from the Grains (Bread, Cereal, Rice & Pasta) group. How does this compare to your spaghetti dinner? Your dinner had 6 servings—the total daily recommendation for someone with your calorie needs. If you had counted your portions of spaghetti and bread as only 1 serving each, you might think you had only eaten 2 servings from the Grains group. But, you actually ate 6! By comparing the portion you ate with a standard Pyramid serving, you can judge whether your daily intake is right for you.
Pyramid serving sizes and the recommended number of servings from each group are guides to help determine your daily intake.

Your portions do not have to match the standard serving size—they can be larger or smaller. But, the amount you eat over the day should match the total amount of a food that is recommended.

Often, the food portions of grains and meats that people choose are larger than the Pyramid serving size.

Portions and servings—What's the difference?

A **portion** is the amount of food you choose to eat. There is no standard portion size and no single right or wrong portion size.

A **serving** is a standard amount used to help give advice about how much to eat or to identify how many calories and nutrients are in a food.

For example: You eat a sandwich with 2 slices of bread. The Food Guide Pyramid **serving size** for bread is 1 slice.

Your **portion** is 2 slices, which equals 2 servings from the Pyramid Grains group.

Your 2 servings are one-third of the Pyramid recommendation of 6 servings for people needing 1,600 calories per day.

How can you follow Pyramid recommendations?

Let's go back to the spaghetti dinner. In this example, you know that you should have 6 daily servings from the Grains group. Before dinner, you estimate that you have already had 3 Grains group servings. So, only 3 more servings would meet your recommended intake.

To keep to 3 servings, you eat only one slice of garlic bread. When you see the large plate of spaghetti, you set aside half on your plate and ask for a "doggie bag" to take it home.

Tips to help you choose sensible portions

When eating out:
• Choose a "small" or "medium" portion. This includes main dishes, side dishes, and beverages as well. Remember that water is always a good option for quenching your thirst.

• If main dish portions are larger than you want, order an appetizer or side dish instead, or share a main dish with a friend.

• Resign from the "clean your plate club"—when you've eaten enough, leave the rest. If you can chill the extra food right away, take it home in a "doggie bag."

• Ask for salad dressing to be served "on the side" so you can add only as much as you want.

• Order an item from the menu instead of the "all-you-can-eat" buffet.

• Once or twice, measure your typical portion of foods you eat often. Use standard measuring cups. This will help you estimate the portion size of these foods and similar foods.

• Be especially careful to limit portions of foods high in calories, such as cookies, cakes, other sweets, and fats, oils, and spreads.

• Try using a smaller plate for your meal.

• Put sensible portions on your plate at the beginning of the meal, and don't take seconds.

Don't be fooled by large portions Many items sold as single portions actually provide 2 or more Pyramid servings. For example, a large bagel may actually be equal to 3 or 4 servings from the Grains group.

A restaurant portion of steak may be more than the recommended amount for the whole day.

Nutrition Facts label serving sizes

The serving sizes listed on the Nutrition Facts label may be different from Food Guide Pyramid serving sizes. Many Pyramid serving sizes are smaller than those on the Nutrition Facts label.

For example, 1 serving of cooked cereal, rice, or pasta is 1 cup for the label but only 1/2 cup for the Pyramid.

Use the Nutrition Facts label to make nutritional comparisons of similar products. *The label serving size is not meant to tell you how much to eat, but to help identify nutrients in a food and to make product comparisons easier.*
To compare the calories and nutrients in two foods, first check the serving size and the number of servings in the package. Serving sizes are provided in familiar units, such as cups or pieces.

The Bottom Line

Choosing sensible portions is a key to controlling calorie intake and getting or keeping your weight in a healthy range.

What is sensible for you?

• Each day, choose the recommended amount from the five Pyramid food groups—depending on your calorie needs.

• A Pyramid serving may not be the same as the portion you choose to eat—compare to find out how many servings are in your portion.

• Keep sensible portions in mind at restaurants as well as at home.

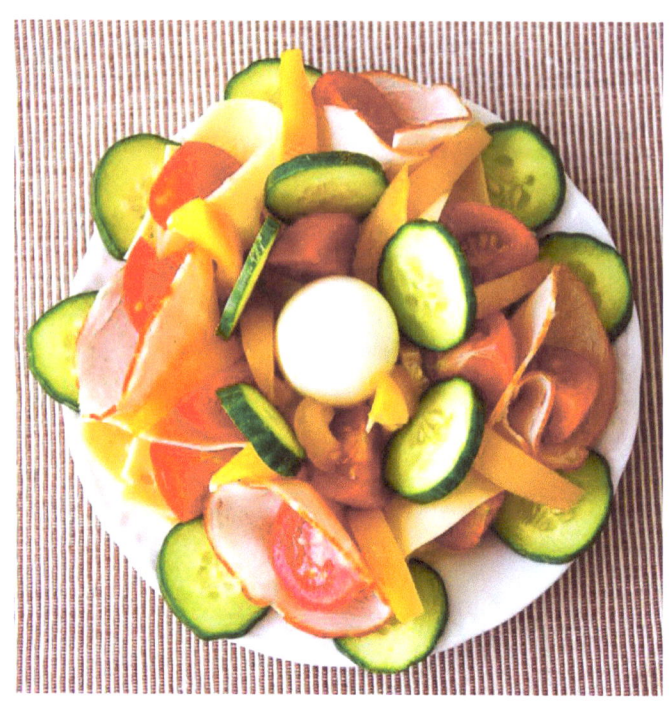

Build a Healthy Plate

Make half your plate fruits and vegetables.

Eat red, orange, and dark-green vegetables, such as tomatoes, sweet potatoes, and broccoli, in main and side dishes.

Eat fruit, vegetables, or unsalted nuts as snacks—they are nature's original fast foods.

Switch to skim or 1% milk.

They have the same amount of calcium and other essential nutrients as whole milk, but less fat and calories.

Try calcium-fortified soy products as an alternative to dairy foods

Make at least half your grains whole.

Choose 100% whole-grain cereals, breads, crackers, rice, and pasta.

Check the ingredients list on food packages to find whole-grain foods.

Vary your protein food choices.

Twice a week, make seafood the protein on your plate.

Eat beans, which are a *natural* source of fiber and protein.

Keep meat and poultry portions small and lean.

Many people eat foods with too much solid fats, added sugars, and salt. (sodium). Added sugars and fats load foods with extra calories you don't need. Too much sodium may increase your blood pressure.

Choose foods and drinks with little or no added sugars.

Drink water instead of sugary drinks. There are about 10 packets of sugar in a 12-ounce can of soda.

Select fruit for dessert. Eat sugary desserts less often.

Choose 100% fruit juice instead of fruit-flavored drinks.

Look out for salt (sodium) in foods you buy it all adds up. Compare sodium in foods like soup, bread, and compare sodium in foods like soup, bread, and frozen meals—and choose the foods with lower numbers.

Add spices or herbs to season food without adding salt.

Eat fewer foods that are high in solid fats.

Make major sources of saturated fats—such as cakes, cookies, ice cream, pizza, cheese, sausages, and hot dogs—occasional choices, not everyday foods.

Select lean cuts of meats or poultry and fat-free or low-fat milk, yogurt, and cheese.

Switch from solid fats to oils when preparing food.*

Examples of solid fats and oils

Solid Fats
Beef, pork, and chicken fat

Butter, cream, and milk fat

Coconut, palm, and palm kernel oils

Hydrogenated oil

Partially hydrogenated oil

Shortening

Stick margarine

Oils
Canola oil

Corn oil

Cottonseed oil

Olive oil

Peanut oil

Safflower oil

Sunflower oil

Tub (soft) margarine and vegetable oil

Everyone has a personal calorie limit. Staying within yours can help you get to or maintain a healthy weight. People who are successful at managing their weight have found ways to keep track of how much they eat in a day, even if they don't count every calorie.

Enjoy your food, but eat less.

Get your personal daily calorie limit at www.ChooseMyPlate.gov and keep that number in mind when deciding what to eat.

Think before you eat…is it worth the calories?

Avoid oversized portions. Use a smaller plate, bowl, and glass. Stop eating when you are satisfied, not full.

Cook more often at home, where *you* are in control of what's in your food.

When eating out, choose lower calorie menu options.

Check posted calorie amounts.

Choose dishes that include vegetables, fruits, and/or whole grains.

Order a smaller portion or share when eating out. Write down what you eat to keep track of how much you eat.

Use food labels to help you make better choices

Most packaged foods have a Nutrition Facts label and an ingredients list. For a healthier you, use this tool to make smart food choices quickly and easily.

Check for calories. Be sure to look at the serving size and how many servings you are actually consuming. If you double the servings you eat, you double the calories.

Choose foods with lower calories, saturated fat, *trans* fat, and sodium.

Check for added sugars using the ingredients list. When a sugar is close to first on the ingredients list, the food is high in added sugars. Some names for added sugars include sucrose, glucose, high fructose corn syrup, corn syrup, maple syrup, and fructose.

Most packaged foods have a Nutrition Facts label and an ingredients list. For a healthier you, use this tool to make smart food choices quickly and easily.

Check for calories. Be sure to look at the serving size and how many servings you are actually consuming. If you double the servings you eat, you double the calories.

Choose foods with lower calories, saturated fat, *trans* fat, and sodium.

Check for added sugars using the ingredients list. When a sugar is close to first on the ingredients list, the food is high in added sugars. Some names for added sugars include sucrose, glucose, high fructose corn syrup, corn syrup, maple syrup, and fructose.

• About 78 million Americans—35 percent of the U.S. adult population ages 20 years or 18older— have pre-diabetes. Pre-diabetes (also called impaired glucose tolerance or impaired fasting glucose) means that blood glucose levels are higher than normal, but not high enough to be called diabetes.

Cancer - Almost one in two men and women— approxi-mately 41 percent of the population—will be 19 diagnosed with cancer during their lifetime.

• Dietary factors are associated with risk of some types of cancer, including breast (post-menopausal), endometrial, colon, kidney, mouth, pharynx, larynx, and esophagus.

Osteoporosis - One out of every two women and one in four men ages. 0 years and older will have an 20 osteoporosis-related fracture in their lifetime.

• About 85 to 90 percent of adult bone mass is acquired by the age of 18 in girls and the age 21of 20 in boys. Adequate nutrition and regular participation in physical activity are important factors in achieving and maintaining optimal bone mass.

Key Terms to Know

Several terms are used throughout *Dietary Guidelines for Americans, 2010* and are essential to understanding the principles and Recommendations discussed:

Calorie Balance. The balance between calories consumed in foods and beverages and calories expended through physical activity and metabolic processes.

Eating Pattern. The combination of foods and beverages that constitute an individual's complete dietary intake over time.

Nutrient Dense. Nutrient-dense foods and beverages provide vitamins, minerals, and other substances that may have positive health effects with relatively few calories. The term "nutrient dense" indicates that the nutrients and other beneficial substances in a food have not been "diluted" by the addition of calories from added solid fats, added sugars, or added refined starches, or by the solid fats naturally present in the food.

Nutrient-dense foods and beverages are lean or low in solid fats, and minimize or exclude added solid fats, sugars, starches, and sodium. Ideally, they also are in forms that retain naturally occurring components, such as dietary fiber.

All vegetables, fruits, whole grains, seafood, eggs, beans and peas, unsalted nuts and seeds, fat-free and low-fat milk and milk products, and lean meats and poultry when

prepared without adding solid fats or sugars—are nutrient-dense foods.

For most Americans, meeting nutrient needs within their calorie needs is an important goal for health. Eating recommended amounts from each food group in nutrient-dense forms is the best approach to achieving this goal and building healthy eating pattern.

Balancing Calories to Manage Weight Achieving
Achieving and sustaining appropriate body weight across the lifespan is vital to maintaining good health and quality of life. Many behavioral, environmental, and genetic factors have been shown to affect a person's body weight. *Calorie balance over time is the key to weight management.*

Calorie balance refers to the relationship between calories consumed from foods and beverages and calories expended in normal body functions (i.e., metabolic processes) and through physical activity. People cannot control the calories expended in metabolic processes, but they can control what they eat and drink, as well as how many calories they use in physical activity.

Calories consumed must equal calories expended for a person to maintain the same body weight. Consuming more calories than expended will result in weight gain. Conversely, consuming fewer calories than expended will result in weight loss. This can be achieved over time by eating fewer calories, being more physically active or, best of all, a combination of the two.

Maintaining a healthy body weight and preventing excess weight gain throughout the lifespan are highly preferable to losing weight after weight gain. Once a person becomes obese, reducing body weight back to a healthy range requires significant effort over a span of time, even years. People who are most successful at losing weight and keeping it off do so through continued attention to calorie balance.

The current high rates of overweight and obesity among virtually all subgroups of the population in the United States demonstrate that many Americans are in *calorie imbalance*—that is, they consume more calories than they expend. To curb the obesity epidemic and improve their health, Americans need to make significant efforts to decrease the total number of calories they consume from foods and beverages and increase calorie expenditure through physical activity.

Achieving these goals will require Americans to select a healthy eating pattern that includes nutrient-dense foods and beverages they enjoy, meets nutrient requirements, and stays within calorie needs. In addition, Americans can choose from a variety of strategies to increase physical activity

Key Recommendations

Prevent and/or reduce overweight and obesity through improved eating and physical activity behaviors.

Control total calorie intake to manage body weight. For people who are overweight or obese, this will mean consuming fewer calories from foods and beverages.

Increase physical activity and reduce time spent in sedentary behaviors. Maintain appropriate calorie balance during each stage of life— childhood, adolescence, adulthood, pregnancy and breastfeeding, and older age.

An Epidemic of Overweight and Obesity

The prevalence of overweight and obesity in the United States is dramatically higher now than it was a few decades ago. This is true for all age groups, including children, adolescents, and adults. One of the largest changes has been an increase in the number of Americans in the obese category. As shown in Table 2-1, the prevalence of obesity has doubled and in some cases tripled between the 1970s and 2008.

The high prevalence of overweight and obesity across the population is of concern because individuals who are overweight or obese have an increased risk of many health problems.

Type 2 diabetes, heart disease, and certain types of cancer are among the conditions most often associated with obesity. Ultimately, obesity can increase the risk of premature death.

These increased health risks are not limited to adults. Weight-associated diseases and conditions that were once diagnosed primarily in adults are now observed in children and adolescents with excess body fat. For example, cardiovascular disease risk factors, such as high blood cholesterol and hypertension, and type II.

Understanding calorie needs

The total number of calories a person needs each day varies depending on a number of factors, including the person's age, gender, height, weight, and level of physical activity. In addition, a desire to lose, maintain, or gain weight affects how many calories should be consumed.

Table 2-3 provides estimated total calorie needs for weight maintenance based on age, gender, and physical activity level. Estimates range from 1,600 to 2,400 calories per day for adult women and 2,000 to 3,000 calories per day for adult men, depending on age and physical activity level. Within each age and gender category, the low end of the range is for sedentary individuals; the high end of the range is for active individuals. Due to reductions in basal metabolic rate that occurs with aging, calorie needs generally decrease for adults as they age.

21

Estimated needs for young children range from 1,000 to 2,000 calories per day, and the range for older children and adolescents varies substantially from 1,400 to 3,200 calories per day, with boys generally having higher calorie needs than girls.

Knowing one's daily calorie needs may be a useful reference point for determining whether the calories that a person eats and drinks are appropriate in relation to the number of calories needed each day. The best way for people to assess whether they are eating the appropriate number of calories is to monitor body weight and adjust calorie intake and participation in physical activity based on changes in weight over time? A calorie deficit of 500 calories or more per day is a common initial goal for weight loss for adults. However, maintaining a smaller deficit can have a meaningful influence on body weight over time.

Source: USDA

Chicken Recipes

Chicken Casserole

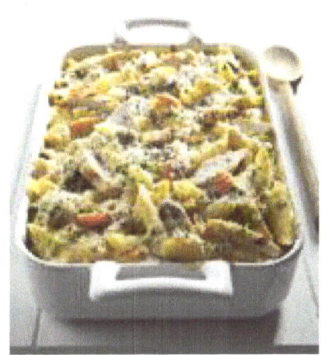

Ingredients

1 tablespoon vegetable oil

2 Chicken breast (whole, skinless, boneless)

1 can diced tomatoes (14 1/2 oz., with juice)

1 cup chili sauce (low sodium)

1 Green Pepper (chopped, large)

2 celery ribs (chopped)

1 onion (chopped, small)

2 garlic clove (minced)

1 teaspoon dried basil

1 teaspoon parsley (dried)

1/4 teaspoon cayenne pepper

1/4 teaspoon salt

Preparation

1. Heat pan over medium-high heat (350 degrees in an electric skillet). Add vegetable oil and chicken and cook until no longer pink when cut (3-5 minutes).
2. Reduce heat to medium (300 degrees in electric skillet).
3. Add tomatoes with juice, chili sauce, green pepper, celery, onion, garlic, basil, parsley, cayenne pepper, and salt.
4. Bring to a boil; reduce heat to low and simmer, covered for 10-15 minutes.
5. Serve over hot, cooked rice or whole wheat pasta.
6. Refrigerate leftovers within 2-3 hours.

3 Cheese Chicken Lasagna

Ingredients

8 lasagna noodles
1/2 c. chopped onion
1/2 c. chopped green pepper
1 can cream of chicken soup
6 oz. sliced mushrooms
1/2 c. chopped pimento, optional
1/2 tsp. crushed basil
1/3 c. milk
1 1/2 c. cottage cheese
2 c. chopped cooked chicken
2 c. shredded American cheese
1/2 c. Parmesan cheese

Preparations

Cook 8 lasagna noodles in boiling water. Drain.
Saute 1/2 cup chopped onion and 1/2 cup chopped
green pepper. Stir in 1 can cream of chicken soup, 6
ounce sliced drained mushrooms, 1/2 cup chopped
pimento, 1/2 teaspoon crushed basil and 1/3 cup
milk.

Place 1/2 of the noodles in 9 x 13 inch baking dish.
Top with 1/2 sauce, 3/4 cup cottage cheese, 1 cup
chopped cooked chicken and 1 cup shredded
American cheese. Repeat all layers and then top
with 1/2 cup Parmesan cheese. Bake at 350 degrees
for about 45 minutes.

Chicken Adobo

Ingredients
Whole chicken, cut-up
1 cup vinegar
1 cup water
4 garlic cloves, crushed
2 bay leaves
1/4 cooking oil
10 peppercorn
1/4 c soy sauce

Preparations

Place chicken and all the ingredients, except oil, in a pot. Cook in medium heat, uncovered, until almost all liquid has evaporated and chicken is cooked. Add cooking oil and fry chicken until brown.
Serve with rice.

Chicken Tostado Salad

Ingredients
16 oz. sour cream
one bag frozen mixed vegetables
1 boiled chicken
1 head shredded lettuce
1 dozen tostada shells

Preparations
1. Boil the chicken, then remove the bones.
2. Cook the mixed vegetables with the chicken pieces.
3. Drain, and add sour cream.

4. Mix with the lettuce.
5. Put it on the tostada shells, and serve.

Chicken Arlette

<u>Ingredients</u>
4 Skinned boned breast halves
4 t butter at room temp
salt and freshly ground pepper
14 oz cheese (cut into four 3/8 inch thick slices)
1/4 c flour
1 egg beaten to blend
2/3 c dry bread crumbs
1/4 c butter
2garlic cloves, finely chopped
1/2c dry white wine.
2t parsley

<u>Preparations</u>

1) Preheat oven to 350 degrees.
2) Place 1 chicken breast between 2 sheets of waxed paper and pound to a thickness of 1/4 inch. Repeat these steps with remaining chicken breasts.
3) Spread one side of pounded chicken with butter, then season with salt and pepper.
4) Top with 1 slice of cheese.
5) Fold chicken over and secure with a toothpick,
6) Roll in flour, dip in beaten egg, then roll in bread crumbs.
7) Transfer chicken to baking dish, seam side down.
8) Melt 1/4c butter, with chopped garlic in small saucepan over low heat til golden brown. Pour over chicken rolls.
9) Bake chicken for 35-40 min.
10) Sprinkle with parsley and serve.

Chicken Fajita Soup

Ingredients
3-4 Chicken Breast
2(14.5 oz.)cans clear chicken broth
1/2 onion chopped
1 toe garlic
2 pks Fajita seasoning
1/2 can Rotel Tomatoes
8 oz. Cheddar Cheese Grated
1 can Cream of Chicken Soup
2 cups Milk
Parsley(to taste)
Corn Starch

Preparations

Put oil in pot and brown chicken. Remove chicken, slice chicken in half into thin strips. Throw in onions and sauté until clear then add garlic, parsley, and sauté no more than 2 minutes. Next, add broth, cream of chicken soup, fajita seasoning, rotel tomatoes, and stir until well blended. Throw in Chicken and cook about 1/2 hour. Thicken with water and corn starch. Eat with brown tortilla chips and put cheddar cheese on top.

Chicken Parmesan

Ingredients

1/4 cup extra-virgin olive oil, plus 3 tablespoons
1 medium onion, chopped
2 garlic cloves, minced
2 bay leaves
1/2 cup kalamata olives, pitted

1/2 bunch fresh basil leaves
2 (28-ounce) cans whole peeled tomatoes, drained
and hand-crushed
Pinch sugar
Kosher salt and freshly ground black pepper
4 skinless, boneless, chicken breasts (about 1-1/2
pounds)
1/2 cup all-purpose flour
2 large eggs, lightly beaten
1 tablespoon water
1 cup dried bread crumbs
1 (8-ounce) ball fresh buffalo mozzarella, water
drained
Freshly grated Parmesan
1 pound spaghetti pasta, cooked al dente

Preparations

Coat a saute pan with olive oil and place over
medium heat. When the oil gets hazy, add the
onions, garlic, and bay leaves; cook and stir for 5
minutes until fragrant and soft. Add the olives and
some hand-torn basil. Carefully add the tomatoes
(nothing splashes like tomatoes), cook and stir until
the liquid is cooked down and the sauce is thick,
about 15 minutes; season with sugar, salt and
pepper. Lower the heat, cover, and keep warm.
Preheat the oven to 450 degrees F.

Get the ingredients together for the chicken so you
have a little assembly line. Put the chicken breasts
side by side on a cutting board and lay a piece of
plastic wrap over them. Pound the chicken breasts
with a flat meat mallet, until they are about 1/2-inch
thick. Put the flour in a shallow platter and season

with a fair amount of salt and pepper; mix with a fork to distribute evenly. In a wide bowl, combine the eggs and water, beat until frothy. Put the bread crumbs on a plate, season with salt and pepper.

Heat 3 tablespoons of olive oil over medium-high flame in a large oven-proof skill Lightly dredge both sides of the chicken cutlets in the seasoned flour, and then dip them in the egg wash to coat completely, letting the excess drip off, then dredge in the bread crumbs. When the oil is nice and hot, add the cutlets and fry for 4 minutes on each side until golden and crusty, turning once.

Ladle the tomato-olive sauce over the chicken and sprinkle with mozzarella, Parmesan, and basil. Bake the Chicken Parmesan for 15 minutes or until the cheese is bubbly. Serve hot with spaghetti

Chicken Parmesan Bake

Ingredients

2 to 3 Pounds of Skinless, Boneless Chicken Tenderloins
1 and 1/2 Cups Mayonnaise
2 Teaspoons of Southwestern Seasoning Mix (*optional)
1 Raw Egg (beaten)
8 Ounces Shredded Parmesan Cheese
1/2 Cup Bread Crumbs

1 (16 ounce) Package of Egg Noodles (cooked as directed)

Optional ~ Oregano, Salt, Pepper or other

favorite seasoning may be used for taste in place of Southwestern Seasoning Mix.

<u>Preparations</u>

Combine mayonnaise, seasoning mix, and egg in large bowl. Mix well. Fold in shredded Parmesan cheese and bread crumbs.
Dip chicken in mixture to coat, place chicken in single layer on non-stick or glass baking dish (cooking spray may be used if needed).
Pour remaining mixture evenly over top of chicken.
Preheat oven to 375 degrees.
Bake chicken for 35-45 minutes or until done.
While chicken is baking, prepared Egg Noodles as directed on package and drain.
Spoon Chicken Parmesan Bake over fully cooked Egg Noodles, and sprinkle with grated Parmesan cheese if desired.
Serve with fresh steamed vegetables and garlic bread.

Chicken with Rice

<u>Ingredients</u>
Rice (make the amount. you usually use but at least one cup less).
4 or 5 small pieces of chicken.
a carrot
food coloring

<u>Preparations</u>

First, make the chicken at your flavor. Then, take the chickens' juice out and let the chicken cool down. After that take the bones out of the chicken and make the chicken into small little pieces. Fourth, make the carrot into small little pieces. Fifth, start making the rice and wait a little while to put the chicken and the carrot. However, do not put salt in it. Sixth, once the rice is ready to put the water instead put the food coloring and the juice left over of the chicken. Lastly, just finish cooking the chicken rice like if it was normal white rice.

Baked Chicken

Ingredients

chicken, boneless, skinless

garlic powder

pepper

Preparations

1. Preheat the oven to 350 degrees.

2. Rinse the chicken.

3. Put the chicken in a baking pan or casserole dish.

4. Sprinkle with garlic powder and pepper to taste.

5. Bake for 1 hour.

Sweet and Sour Chicken

Ingredients

4 to 6 Oz. Lean Boneless Chicken
Peanut Oil for Deep Frying.

BATTER:
1 egg
1/3 cup milk
½ cup flour
½ tsp. baking powder

SAUCE:
2/3 cup sugar
2 Tbsp. rice vinegar
3 Tbsp. ketchup
¾ cup water
2 Tbsp. cornstarch

Preparations

Mix all sauce ingredients in saucepan. Stir over
medium heat until sauce thickens

Dip meat in batter and deep fry until done. Set
aside. Dip in sauce or pour over meat.

Tandoori Chicken

Ingredients
Chicken
1 lb boneless chicken cut into about 1" cubes
1 TB chicken masala
2 TB plain yogurt
1/4 tsp garam maschiala
1 TB lemon juice
1 TB oil
1/4 tsp. salt
1/4 tsp. coriander, ground
1 clove garlic, minced
1 small piece ginger, minced

Indian Rice
(I double this, too. The leftovers are grand.)
1 C Basmati rice
2 C water
1 tsp cumin seed
1 small onion (I use large)
1 TB oil

Cilantro Chutney (Fabulous!)
1 bunch cilantro
1 small onion
2 TB lemon juice (I prefer lime)
1/2 tsp salt
1-5 jalapeno peppers (1 is enough for me.)
(I love to add 1 small piece of ginger, too)

Preparations

Chicken
Mix all ingredients in large container. Keep in
refrigerator for at least 3 hours. Oil a large skillet

(We use an electric roaster. A wok would work.), and cook the chicken mix on high heat for about 5 minutes, stirring constantly. Turn heat to med. and cover, cooking for another 5-8 minutes or until thoroughly cooked. Serve over rice (or in pita bread), and with green chutney (recipes below).

Rice

Wash rice 2-3 times. Soak 15-20 minutes. Cut onion in long pieces. Put oil in large pot and heat. Add cumin seeds, then onions, and let it brown. (I like to do this on medium heat, so the onions carmelize a little--awesome!) Add water and rice, bring to boil. Turn heat to medium, cover pot halfway. After 5 minutes, cover pot and cook for 5-8 minutes. Turn heat off and let stand for next 10-15 minutes.

Cilantro Chutney
Wash cilantro and cut into pieces. Peel onion and cut into pieces. Blend all in blender or food processor until smooth. (Optional, instead of cilantro, use mint or a mix of the two.)

Granny's Italian Chicken

Ingredients

(1)family pack chicken wings
(1)16 ounce Italian dressing
(1)bellpepper
(1)onion
11 inch pan
Creole seasoning

Preparations

1.)Cut up pepper and onion.
2.)Clean and season your chicken.
3.)Place chicken in pan and add your Italian dressing on top.
4.)Place aluminum foil on top of pan, put in the oven at 350 degrees,let cook for 25min. covered;remove foil and continue to let it cook until golden brown.

Pearlu Rice (Chicken and Ham in a Stew)

Ingredients
1 3-lb. chicken
salt
pepper
paprika
1 cup cooking oil
2 lbs. oven ready ham
1 cup onions, chopped coarsely
2 cups cabbage, chopped coarsely
2 quarts water
1 6-oz. can tomato paste
1 Tbs. salt
1 tsp. black pepper
few drops tabasco
2 cups uncooked brown rice

Preparations

Cut 1 3-lb. chicken in 8 serving pieces. Wash, drain, and dry.
Spread out and allow to stand for 15 minutes. Dip in flour seasoned with salt, pepper,and paprika.
In a 9-inch heavy skillet: Brown chicken in 1 cup cooking oil, on all sides. Transfer to a 6-quart Dutch oven or heavy pot.

Brown 2 lbs.oven ready ham cut in 1-inch cubes on all sides, in the same skillet.
Add to the pot: 1 cup onions, chopped coarsely and 2 cups cabbage, chopped coarsely.

Blend 2 quarts water, 1 6-oz. can tomato paste, 1 Tbs. salt, 1 tsp. black pepper and a few drops tabasco.
Add the liquid to the pot. Simmer covered for 30 minutes. Remove chicken from the pot. Add 2 cups uncooked
brown rice. Cook for 45 minutes, adding water if necessary during cooking.

Return chicken to pot about 5 minutes before ready to serve.

Easy Cheesy Stuff Chicken

Ingredients
2 Tbsp.butter or margarine
2 medium zucchini, shredded (about 2 cups)
1 medium onion, chopped
1 pkg.(6 0z).Stove Top Stuffing Mix for Chicken
1 cup Kraft Finely Shredded Italian Style Five Cheese Blend
2 pkg.(about 1-2 lb.each) Chicken quarters
3/4 cup Kraft Honey Barbecue Sauce

Preparations

Prep:30 min. | Total:1 hour 25min.

PREHEAT oven to 400 degrees F. Melt butter in medium saucepan on medium heat. Add zucchini and onion; cook and stir 2 min. or until well blended.

CAREFULLY insert fingers between the meat and skin of each chicken quarter to form a pocket. Fill pockets evenly with stuffing mixture. Place, skin sides up, in large roasting pan.

BAKE 45 min. or until chicken is cooked through. Brush with barbecue sauce. Bake an additional 5 to 10 min.or until heated though.

Sesame Chicken

Ingredients
3 whole boneless chicken breasts
Marinade:
2 tablespoons light soy sauce
1 tablespoon cooking wine or dry sherry a few drops of sesame oil
2 tablespoons flour
2 tablespoons cornstarch
2 tablespoons water 1/4 teaspoon baking powder
1/4 teaspoon baking soda
1 teaspoon vegetable oil
Sauce for Sesame Chicken: 1/2 cup water
1 cup chicken broth
1/8 cup vinegar 1/4 cup cornstarch
1 cup sugar
2 TB dark soy sauce
2 TB sesame oil
1 tsp chili paste, or more if desired
1 clove garlic (minced)
2 tablespoons toasted sesame seeds
3 1/2 - 4 cups peanut oil for deep-frying.

Preparations

Toast the sesame seeds and set aside.
Cut the chicken into 1-inch cubes. Mix the
marinade ingredients and marinate the chicken for
20 minutes.
To prepare the sauce: mix together all of the sauce
ingredients. Pour them into a small pot and bring to
a boil, stirring continuously.
Turn the heat down to low and keep warm while
you are deep-frying the chicken.
Turn the heat down to low and keep warm while
you are deep-frying the chicken.
To deep-fry the chicken: add the marinated chicken
pieces a few at a time, and deep-fry until golden
brown. Drain on paper towels. Repeat with the
remainder of the chicken.

Just before you are finished deep-frying, bring the
sauce back up to a boil.

Place the chicken on a large platter and pour the
sauce over. Sprinkle with sesame seeds. Serve the
Sesame Chicken with rice.

Chicken Salad Sandwich

<u>Ingredients</u>

Quick chicken salad sandwich recipe

- 2 c. cooked chicken, chopped (canned is OK)
- ¼ c. onion (red), minced
- ¼ c. sliced celery
- ¼ c. carrots, diced
- 1 Tbsp. chopped fresh dill
- ⅓ c. mayo
- Salt and ground black pepper
- 4 roughly torn leaves of green lettuce leaf
- 2 sliced Roma tomatoes
- 1 package of dinner rolls

For the plain chicken salad sandwich recipe:

1. Place chicken, celery, carrots (peeled and finely diced), onion, dill and mayonnaise in a medium bowl. Stir until the ingredients are combined. Sprinkle with salt and pepper to taste.
2. Cut the rolls in half.
3. Add the tomato and lettuce to the bottom half of rolls.
4. Top with the chicken mixture, and then add the top bun.

Chicken salad made with cream cheese

Make most of the ingredients the same way you did before except:

1. Melt ¼ cup of cream cheese in the microwave or leave out at room temperature until it's soft.
2. Add the cream cheese to ¼ cup of mayonnaise.
3. Season with salt, pepper, paprika, and garlic powder to taste.
4. Place it on homemade bread

Chicken Salad Classics

Ingredients

1 package of long grain and wild rice - (Near East preferred) cooked according to directions on the package
* 3 cups of chicken - cooked and cut into chunks
* 3 green onions - chopped
* 1 red bell pepper - diced
* 1/3 cup of your favorite vinaigrette dressing
* 1 lemon - juiced
* 2 medium avocados - chopped
* 1/2 cup of pecans

Preparations

Mix together cooked rice, cooked chicken, chopped scallions, and diced red pepper and salad dressing. Refrigerate until ready to serve.

Before serving, peel and chop avocados. Pour the lemon juice over the avocados to coat.

Add just the avocados to the salad. Serve on lettuce leaves and garnish with pecans.

Stuffed Chicken Breast

Ingredients

Chicken Breast
Mozzarella Slice

Spinach (stems removed)

bread crumbs (unseasoned)

chicken seasoning (I used Morton's)

Pepper

Preparations

Pound chicken breast down to a flat, even thickness. Try to get it relatively thin as you'll be rolling the chicken later.

1. Season both sides with the chicken seasoning and pepper.
2. Add bread crumbs to both sides and press into the chicken
3. lay the chicken on a baking dish and pre-heat the oven to 375 degrees
4. Add the spinach on to the chicken breast creating a single layer across all of the chicken

5. layer on top of the spinach a mozzarella slice. You may need to tear the slice into pieces for even distribution
6. Carefully roll the chicken and tie or pin it together
7. Cook for 20-25 minutes and then cut and serve

Chicken Caesar Wrap

<u>Ingredients</u>

1pc Tortilla

- 100gr Chicken breast
- 100gr Lettuce Iceberg
- 25gr Mayonnaise
- 10gr Parmesan cheese (ground)

Marinated

- Chicken breast
- Little bit olive oil
- Pinch of salt and pepper

<u>Preparations</u>

Marinated chicken and bake in moderate oven with steam for 25 minutes and 200C.

1. Remove from the oven, rest for a while time after that chop the chicken and mix with mayonnaise and Parmesan cheese. Last of fold it tight with tortilla.
2. Serve it and enjoy cold.

Although this is the end of The Calorie Count Method Guide book with delicious chicken recipes, let this be the beginning of a successful weight management journey…

www.ingramcontent.com/pod-product-compliance
Lightning Source LLC
Chambersburg PA
CBHW050839290526
45792CB00001B/459

* 9 7 8 1 4 8 4 9 1 8 8 4 5 *